reading room

red hall

bathroom

guest room 2

kitchen

mud/linens room

Floor

Obscura the Cat Sees Beyond

Ben Franchi

Illustrated by Cheyenne Bigham

BROWN BOOKS KIDS

Obscura the Cat Sees Beyond

Brown Books Kids
Dallas / New York
www.BrownBooksKids.com
(972) 381-0009

A New Era in Publishing®

Names: Franchi, Ben, author. | Bigham, Cheyenne, illustrator.
Title: Obscura the cat sees beyond / Ben Franchi ; illustrated by Cheyenne Bigham.
Description: Dallas ; New York : Brown Books Kids, [2023] | Interest age level: 006-010. | Summary: You're
    in for a thrill as Obscura the Cat Sees Beyond! Obscura avoids the ghosts and the ghouls that refuse to
    leave her alone As the end nears, will she face her fears and vanquish her haunted home? Join the not-
    so-feisty feline as she navigates her haunted house in search of her owners, encountering all manner of
    spooky sights along the way.--Publisher.
Identifiers: ISBN: 978-1-61254-565-3 (hardcover) | 978-1-61254-617-9 (ePub) | LCCN: 2023932210
Subjects: LCSH: Cats--Juvenile fiction. | Haunted houses--Juvenile fiction. | Cat owners--Juvenile fiction.
    | Courage--Juvenile fiction. | Intellect--Juvenile fiction. | CYAC: Cats--Fiction. | Ghosts--Fiction.
    | Haunted houses--Fiction. | Cat owners--Fiction. | Courage--Fiction. | Intellect--Fiction. | LCGFT:
    Ghost stories. | BISAC: JUVENILE FICTION / Animals / Cats. | JUVENILE FICTION / Paranormal,
    Occult & Supernatural. | JUVENILE FICTION / Holidays & Celebrations / Halloween.
Classification: LCC: PZ7.1.F734 Ob 2023 | DDC: [E]--dc23

ISBN 978-1-61254-565-3
LCCN 2023932210

Printed in China
10 9 8 7 6 5 4 3 2 1

For more information or to contact the author, please go to
www.BenFranchi.com.

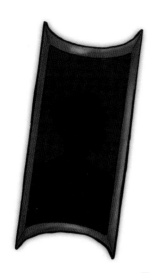
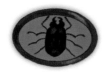
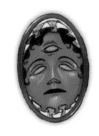

Dedication

To all the weird and wonderful pets out there,
and all the good you do for your strange and silly owners.

Acknowledgments

I would like to thank my mom, dad, and my sister for supporting my passions and the pursuit of my dreams. I would like to thank Cheyenne for the brilliant illustrations you've provided for this book. I would like to thank Brown Books for providing the opportunity and guidance to see this work become a reality. I would like to thank Morgan for bringing Cherry home and for being a reliable friend. I would like to thank Renna for her endless support and keeping my headspace in check. I would like to thank Cherry, the cat, whom the existence of this book to begin with has her to thank.

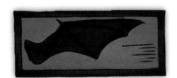
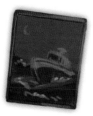
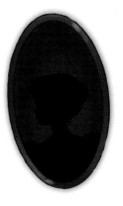

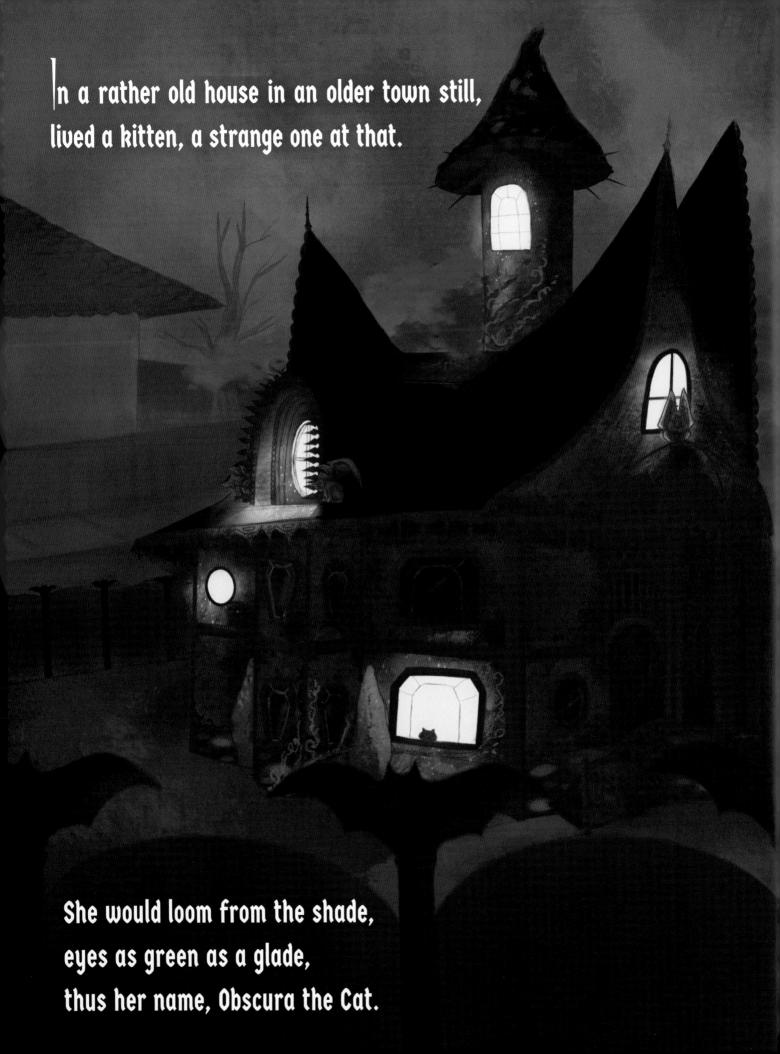

In a rather old house in an older town still,
lived a kitten, a strange one at that.

She would loom from the shade,
eyes as green as a glade,
thus her name, Obscura the Cat.

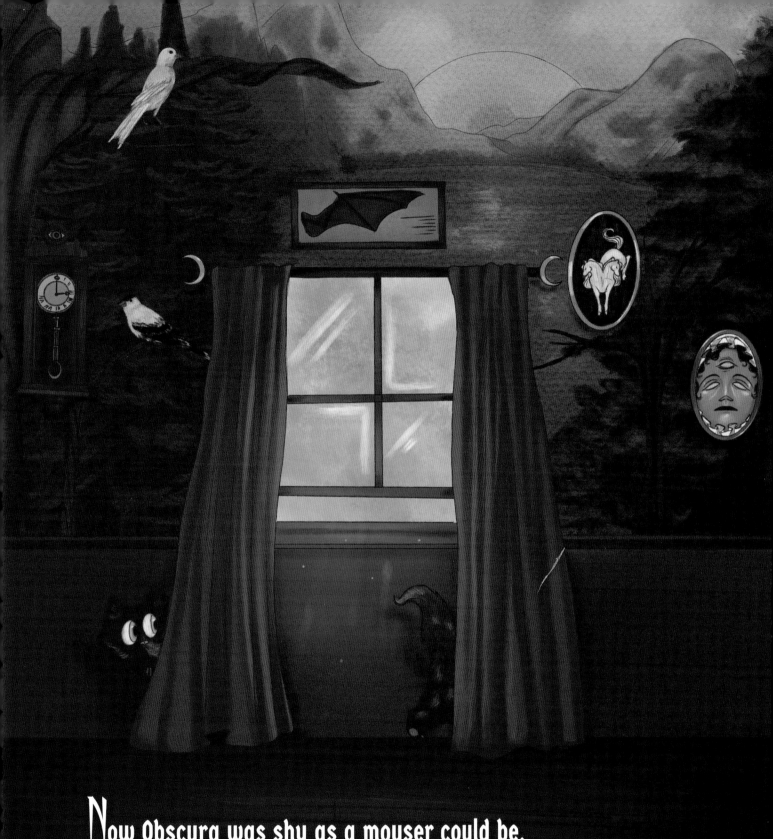

Now Obscura was shy as a mouser could be,
no one ever caught her when she roamed.
She was silent and scared, making not but a peep,
since she moved to this ancient new home.

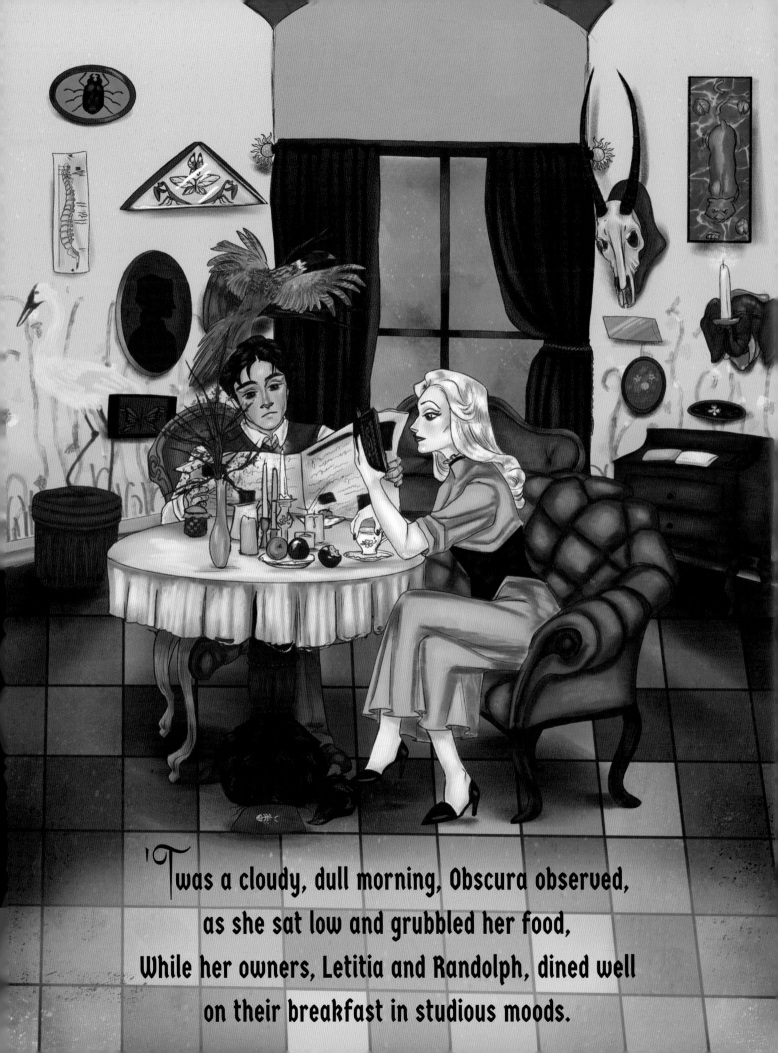

'Twas a cloudy, dull morning, Obscura observed,
as she sat low and grubbled her food,
While her owners, Letitia and Randolph, dined well
on their breakfast in studious moods.

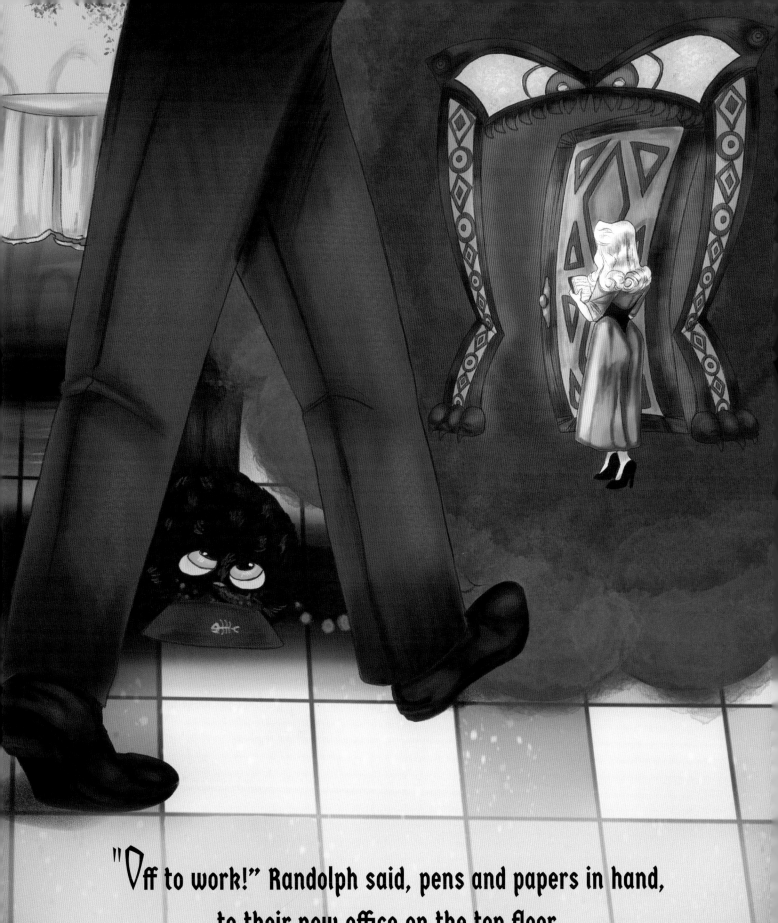

"Off to work!" Randolph said, pens and papers in hand,
to their new office on the top floor.
A mysterious place that Obscura knew not,
never crossing its thick wooden door.

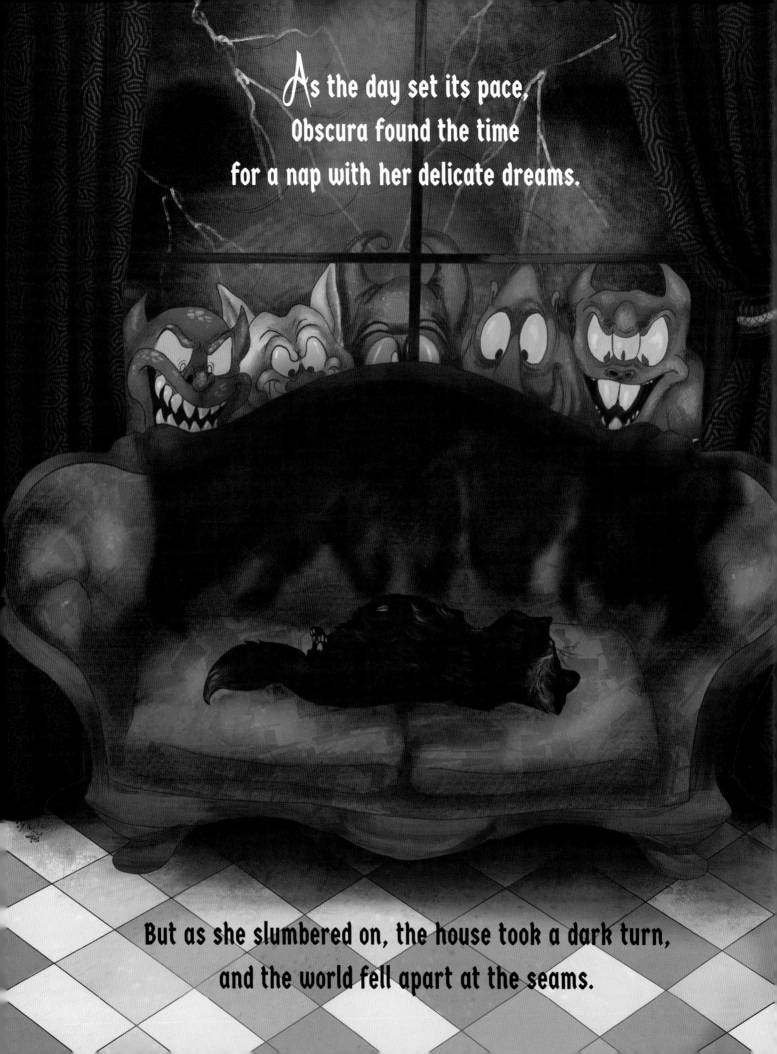

As the day set its pace,
Obscura found the time
for a nap with her delicate dreams.

But as she slumbered on, the house took a dark turn,
and the world fell apart at the seams.

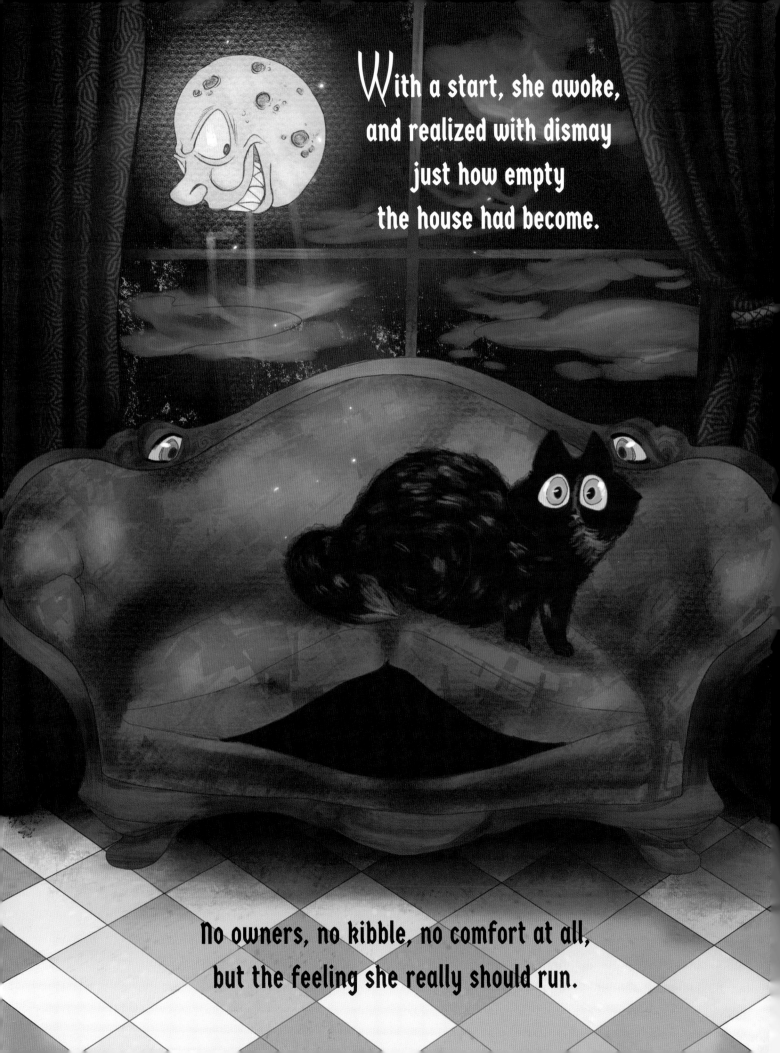

And run fast she did, for the chairs sprung to life,
and the table reared up quite tall!
Around in a lap, they galloped and clapped,
and chased her down the long hall.

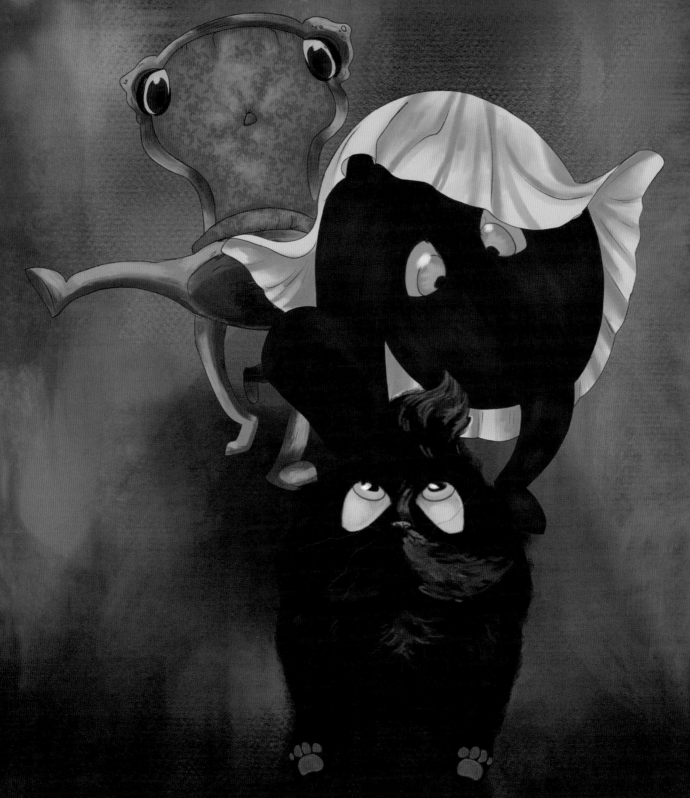

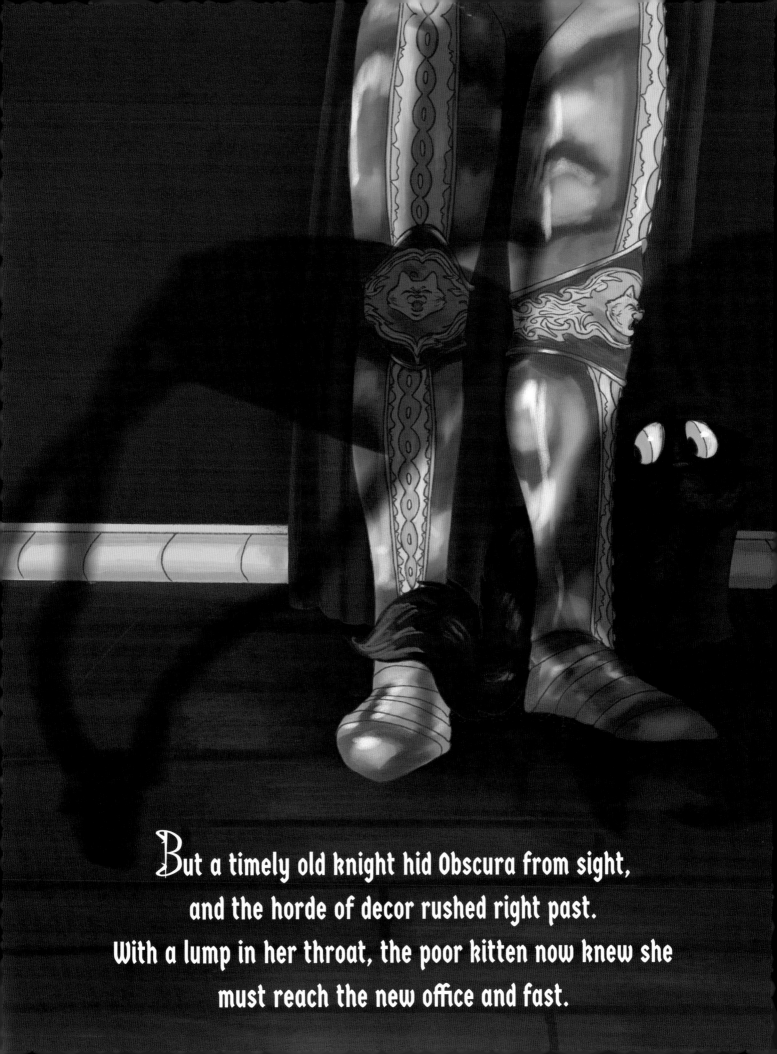

But a timely old knight hid Obscura from sight,
and the horde of decor rushed right past.
With a lump in her throat, the poor kitten now knew she
must reach the new office and fast.

An assortment of ghouls, freaks, and creeps of all kinds
marched about in a monsterous parade.
Yet they didn't quite catch that Obscura could match
the wallpaper's particular shade.

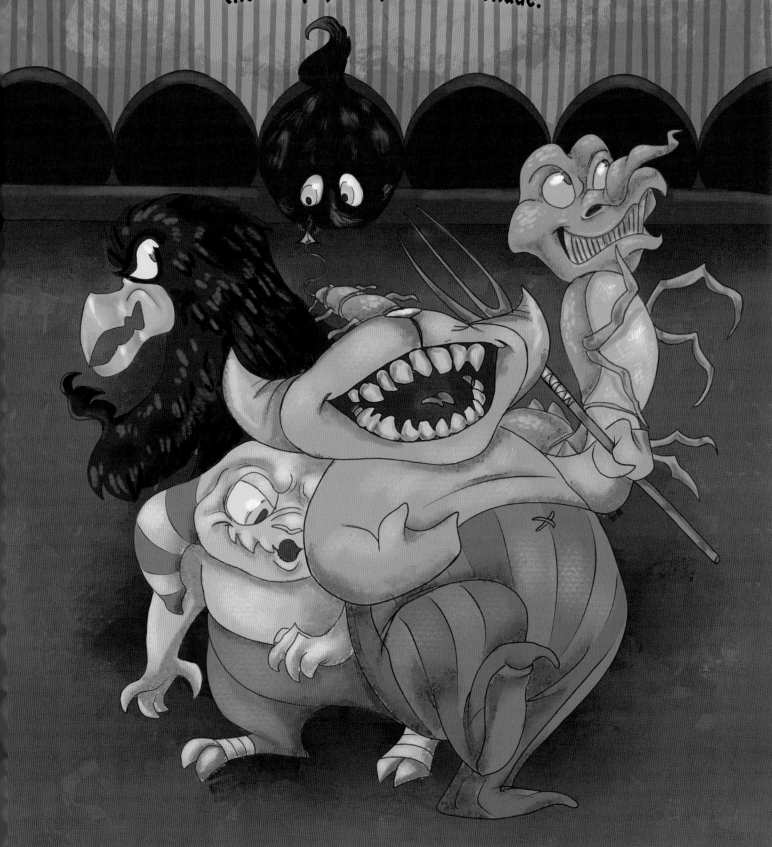

The smell of fine food and most savory meats
drew Obscura to the kitchen's light.
But the chuckling Boney Boys cooking the stew
frightened her clear out of sight.

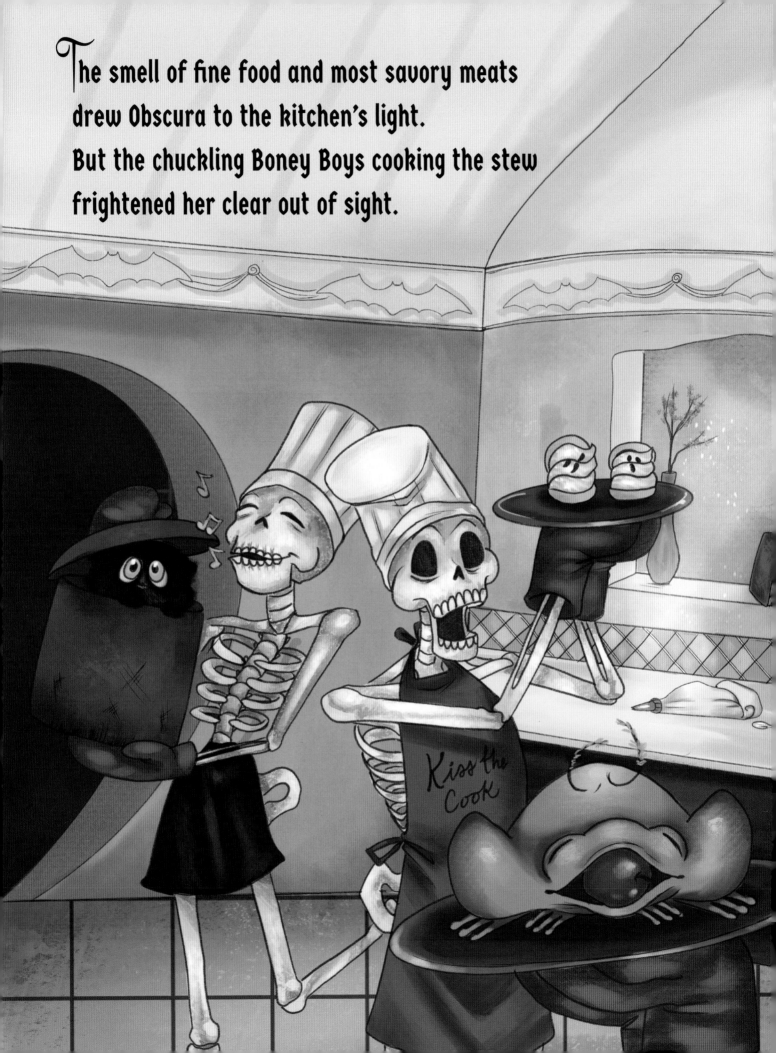

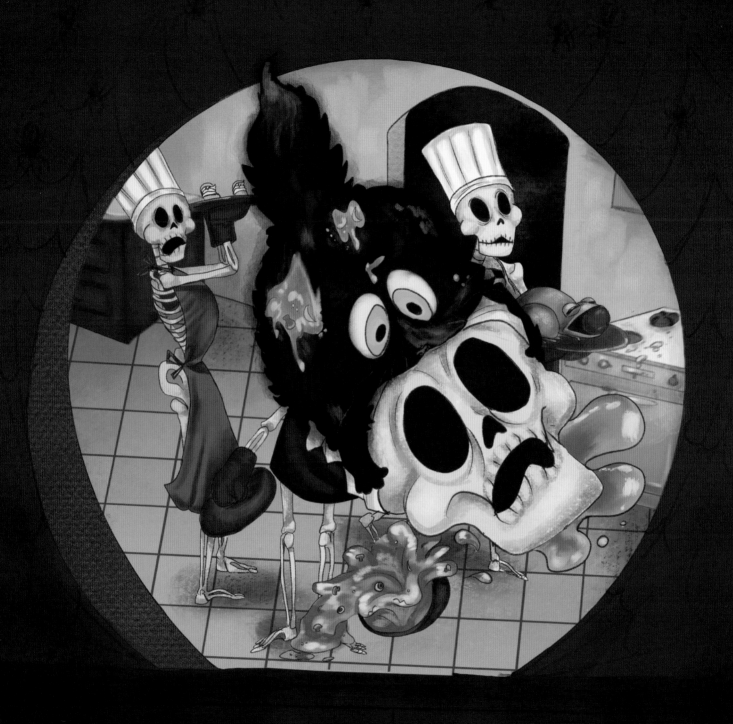

As the Boys cackled on, Obscura peeped outside;
the chef prepared his dishes to taste.
She sprung through the air, gave the cacklers a scare,
and scurried to the bathroom in haste.

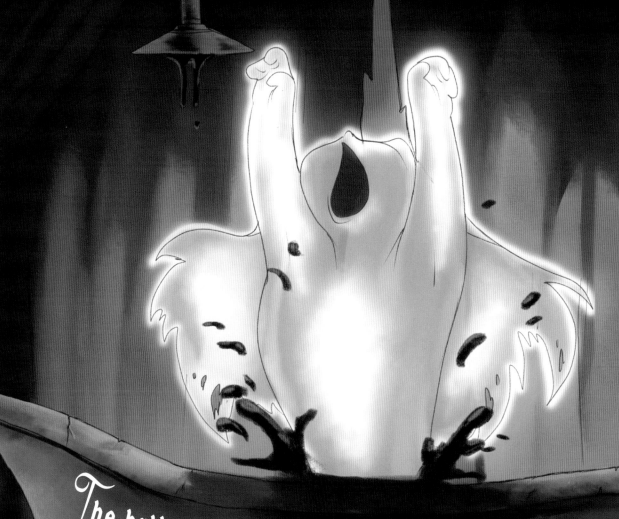

The bathroom was far from a welcoming place;
'twas quite cold and so terribly dark.
But worse was the shade of old Agatha Cree
who rose up screaming,

"HARK".

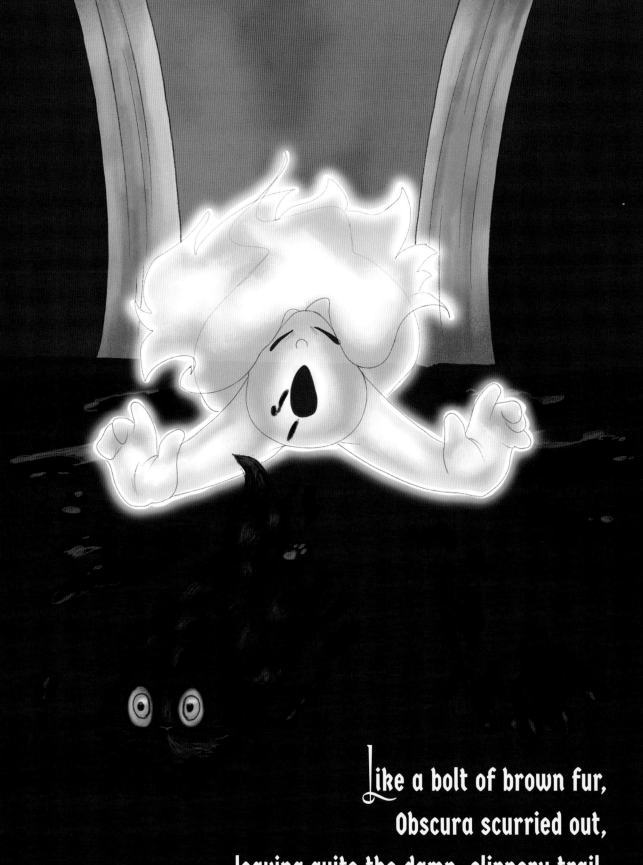

Like a bolt of brown fur,
Obscura scurried out,
leaving quite the damp, slippery trail.
As ol' Cree took pursuit, she slipped on the wet floor,
falling back with a screech and a flail.

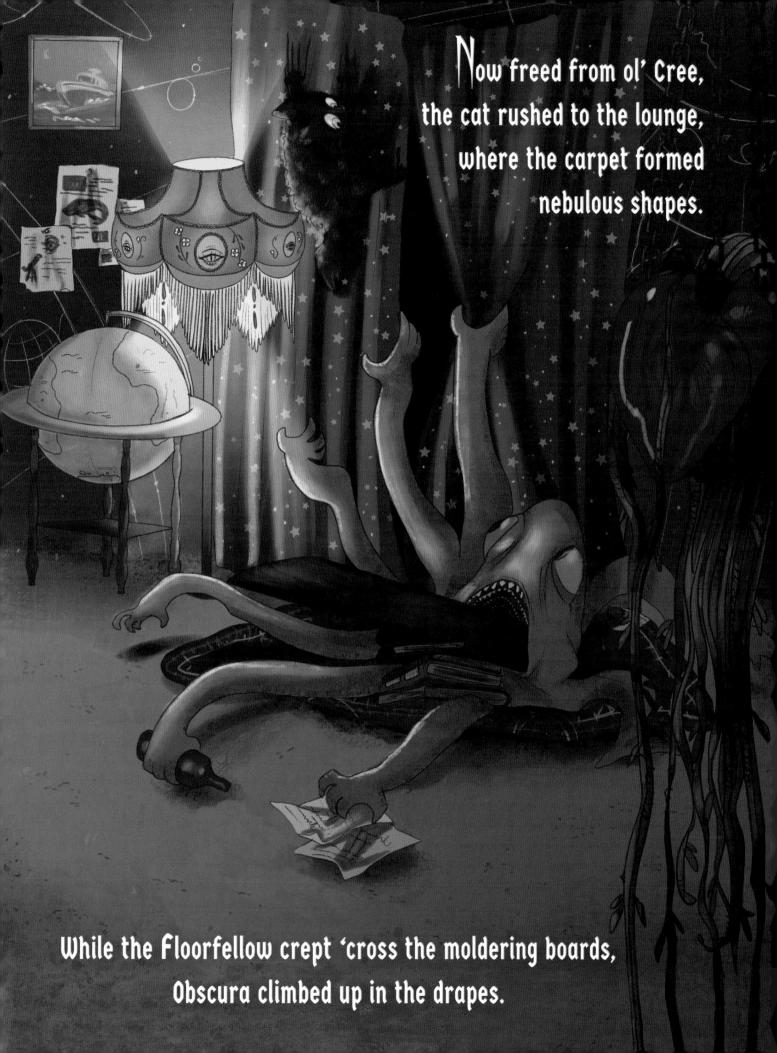

Now freed from ol' Cree,
the cat rushed to the lounge,
where the carpet formed
nebulous shapes.

While the Floorfellow crept 'cross the moldering boards,
Obscura climbed up in the drapes.

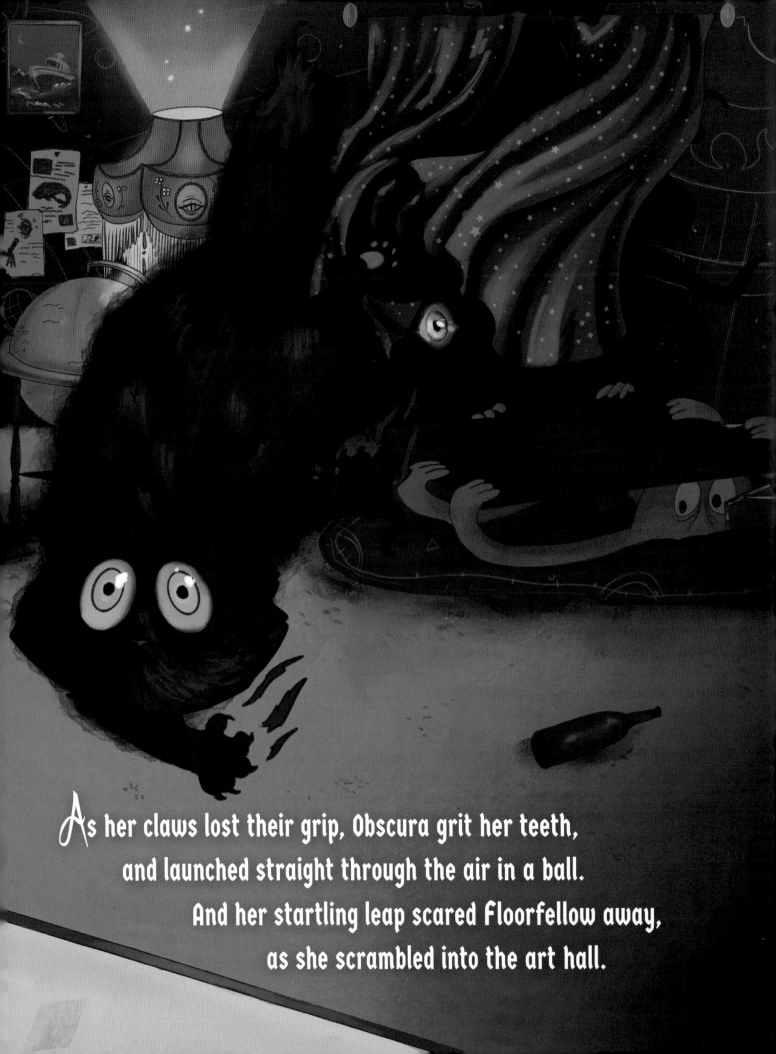

As her claws lost their grip, Obscura grit her teeth,
and launched straight through the air in a ball.
And her startling leap scared Floorfellow away,
as she scrambled into the art hall.

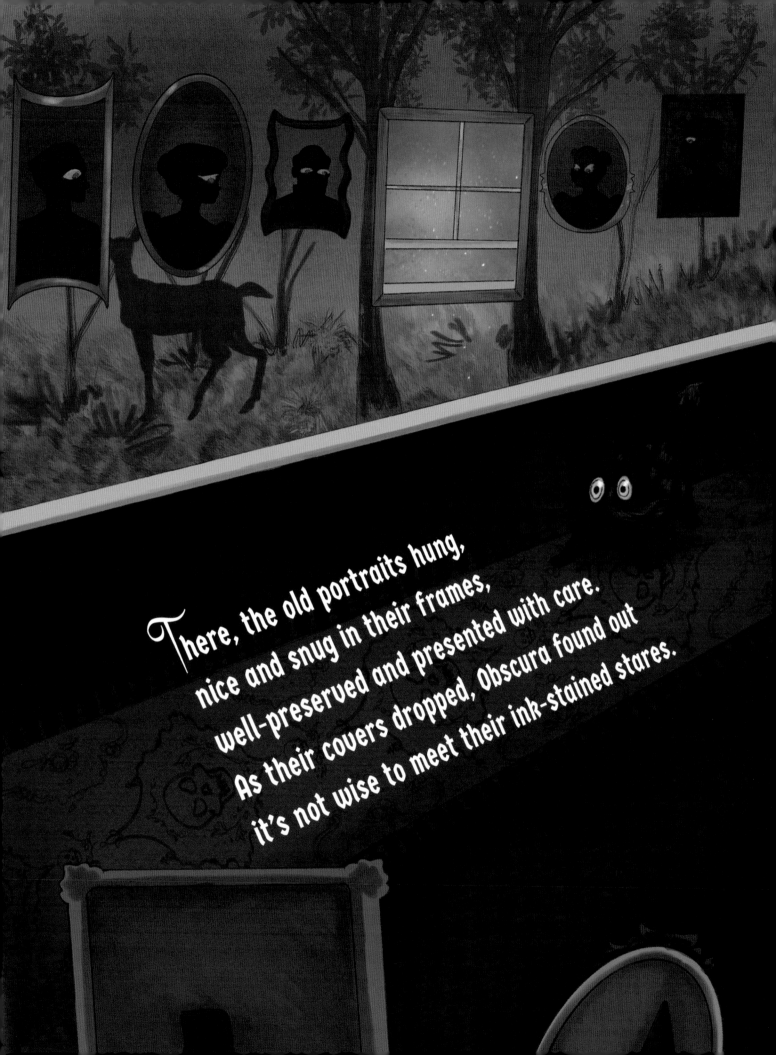

There, the old portraits hung,
nice and snug in their frames,
well-preserved and presented with care.
As their covers dropped, Obscura found out
it's not wise to meet their ink-stained stares.

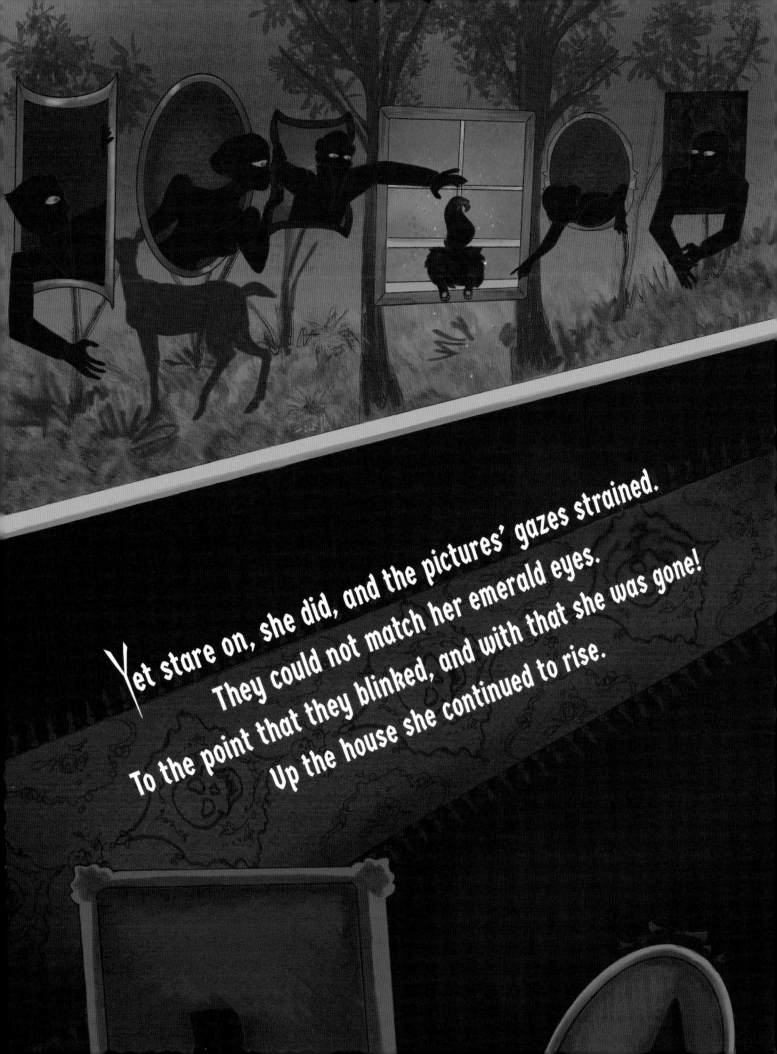

Yet stare on, she did, and the pictures' gazes strained.
They could not match her emerald eyes.
To the point that they blinked, and with that she was gone!
Up the house she continued to rise.

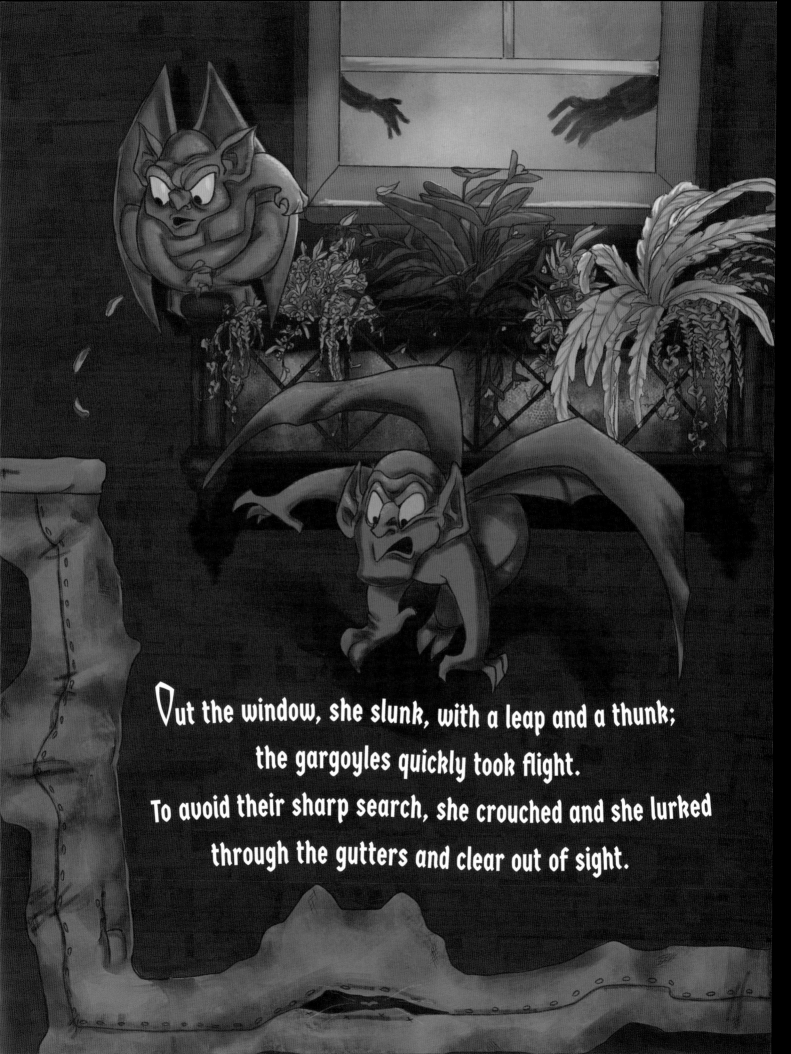

Out the window, she slunk, with a leap and a thunk;
the gargoyles quickly took flight.
To avoid their sharp search, she crouched and she lurked
through the gutters and clear out of sight.

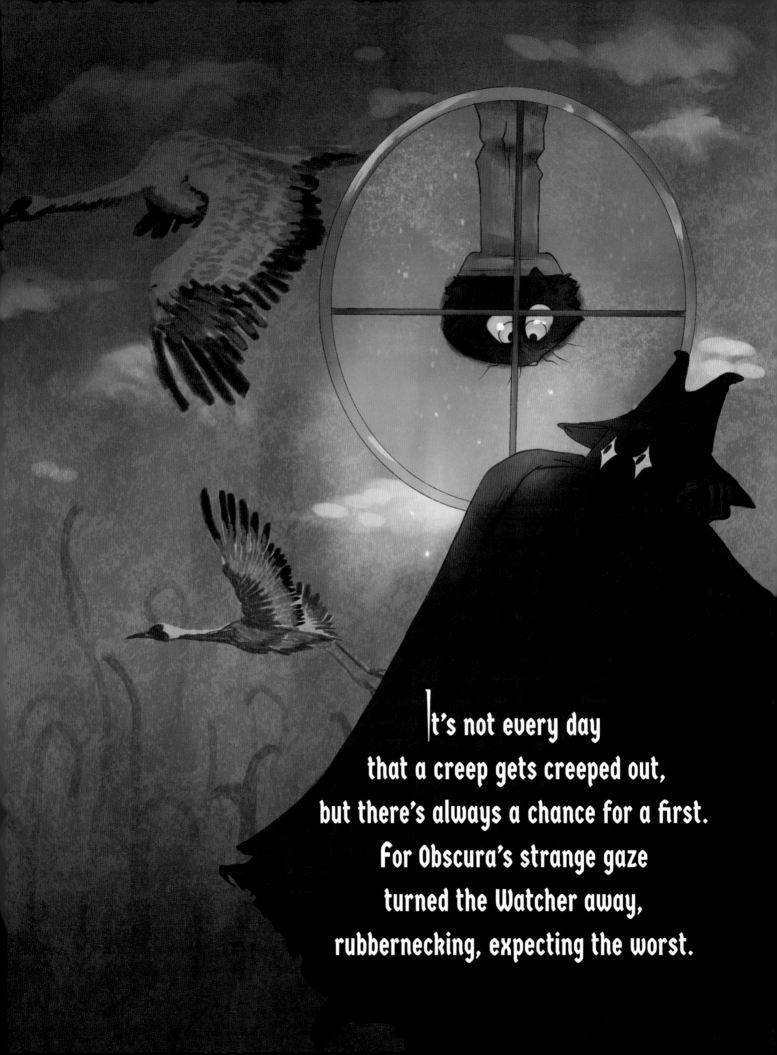

It's not every day
that a creep gets creeped out,
but there's always a chance for a first.
For Obscura's strange gaze
turned the Watcher away,
rubbernecking, expecting the worst.

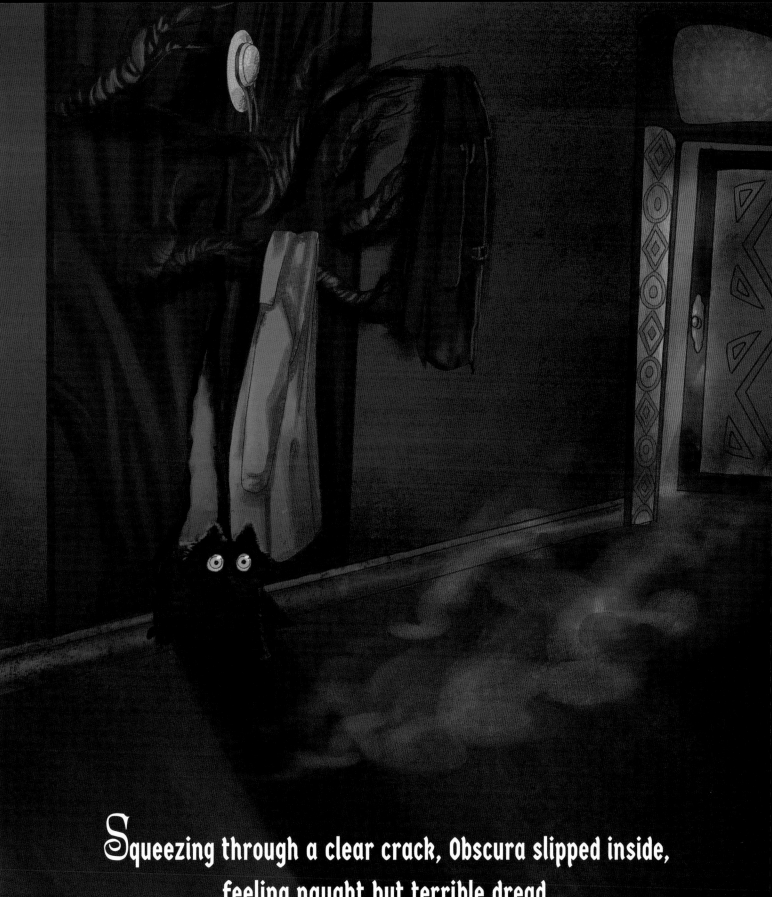

Squeezing through a clear crack, Obscura slipped inside,
feeling naught but terrible dread.
But the end was in sight, for beyond the oak door,
the office lay just ahead.

Something creaked, something moaned, something shook
the old stones, and the house's dark spirit took shape.
The cat froze in place as the Hearth came to life,
blocking her only escape.

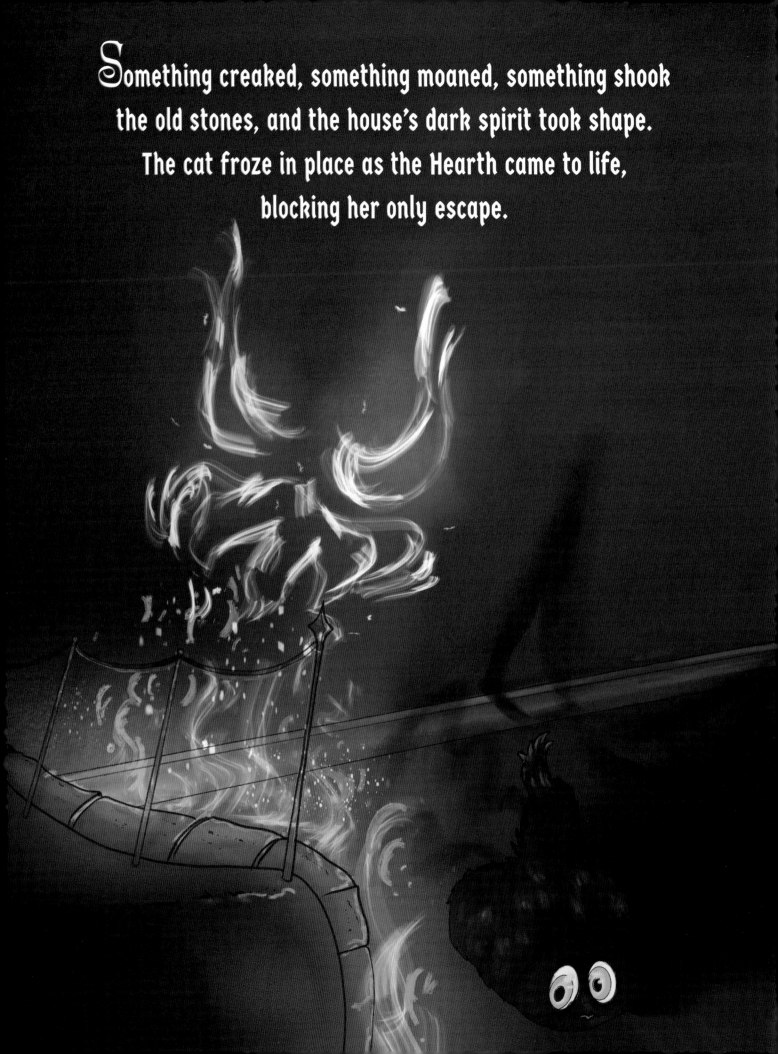

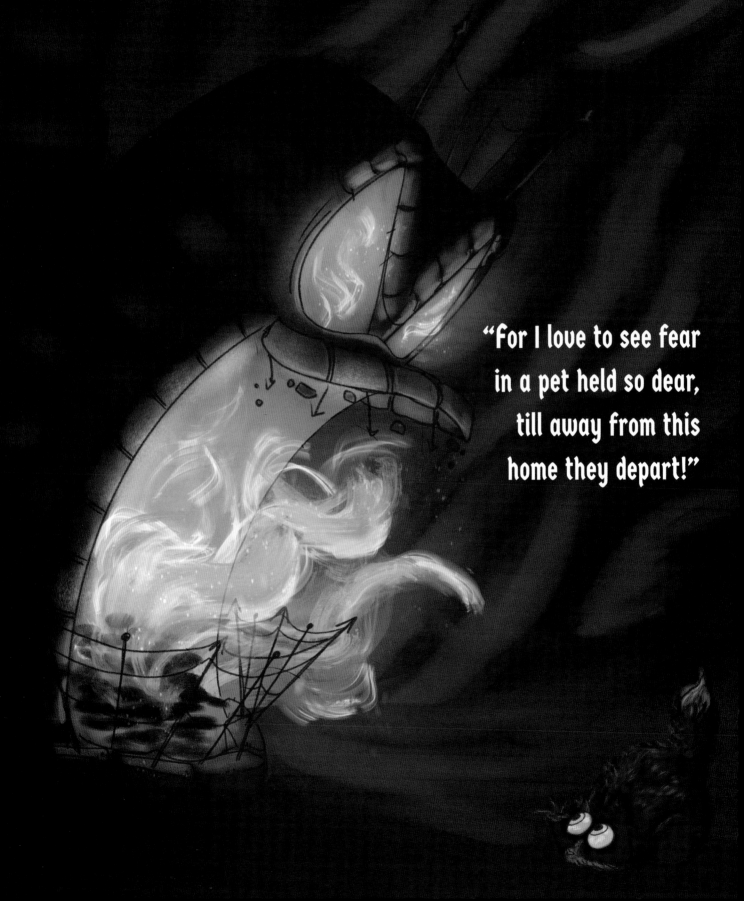

"Do you cower, small cat?" the Hearth bellowed quite loud.
"I should hope so, it warms my black heart!

"For I love to see fear
in a pet held so dear,
till away from this
home they depart!"

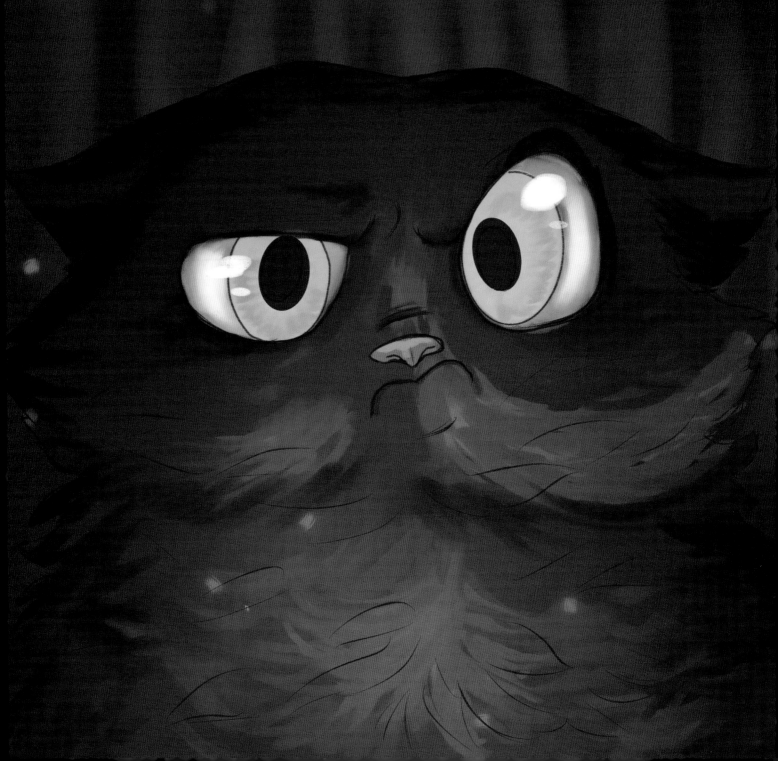

But Obscura had made it this long and this far,
through her guts and her guile and her will.
Drawing up her full height, she locked eyes with the Hearth;
for the first time, its bricks felt a chill.

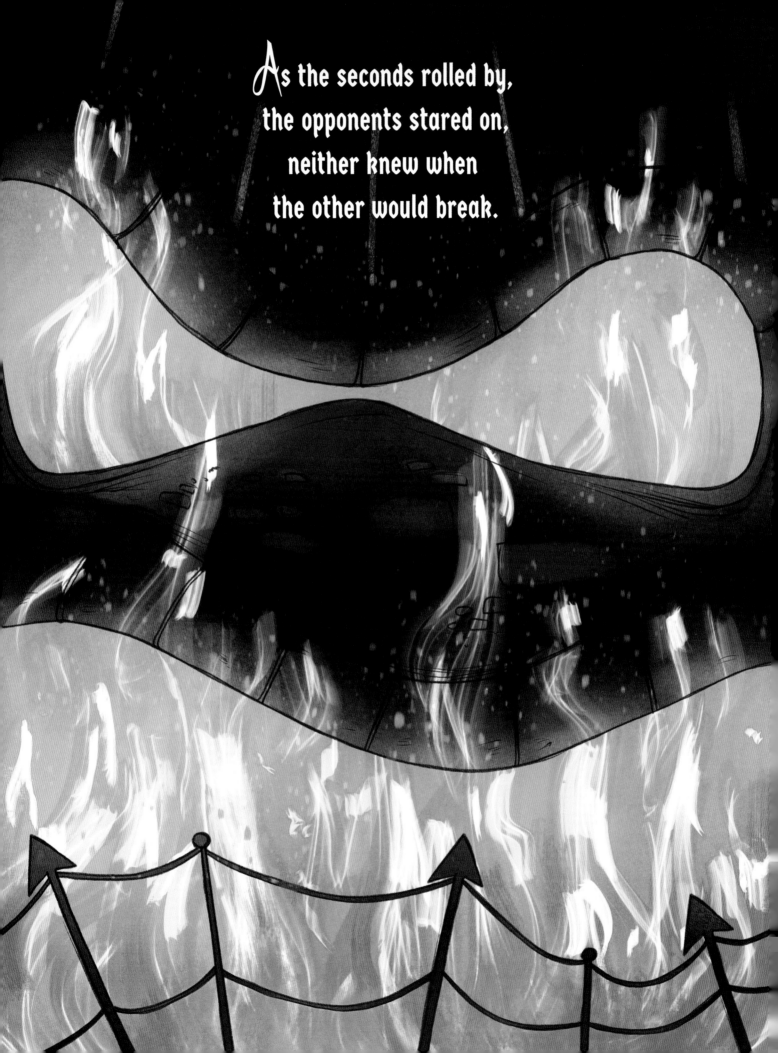

As the seconds rolled by,
the opponents stared on,
neither knew when
the other would break.

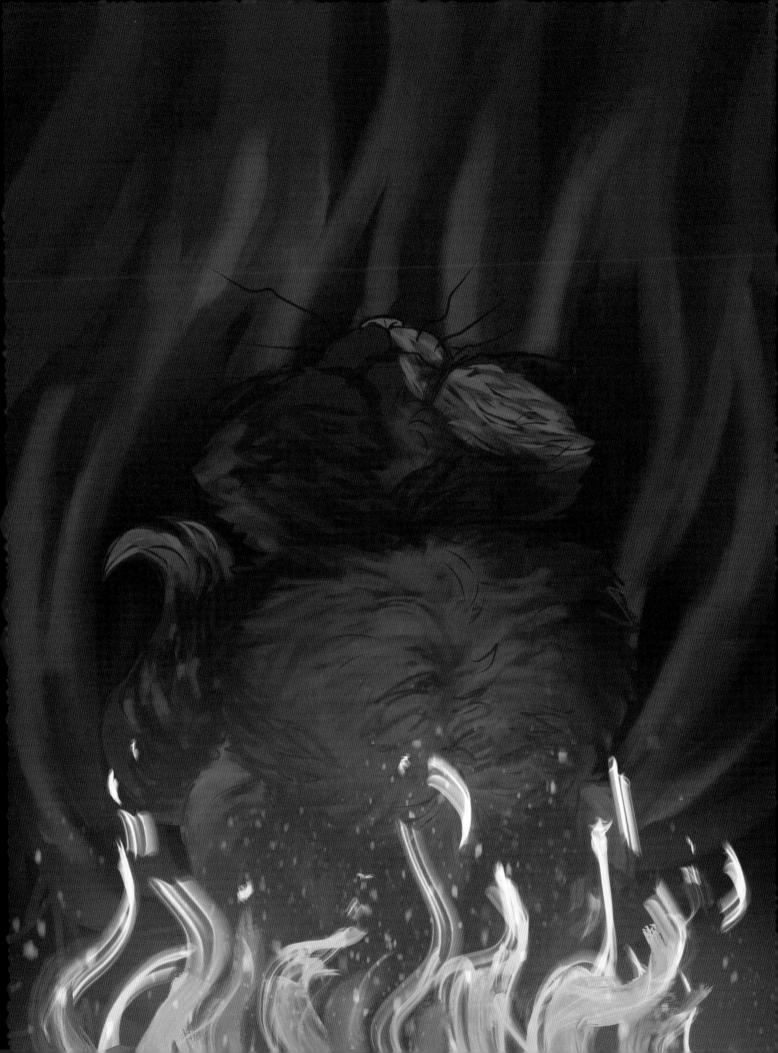

Then the stony wraith blinked, and Obscura rushed forth, with the mightiest **MEOW** she could make!

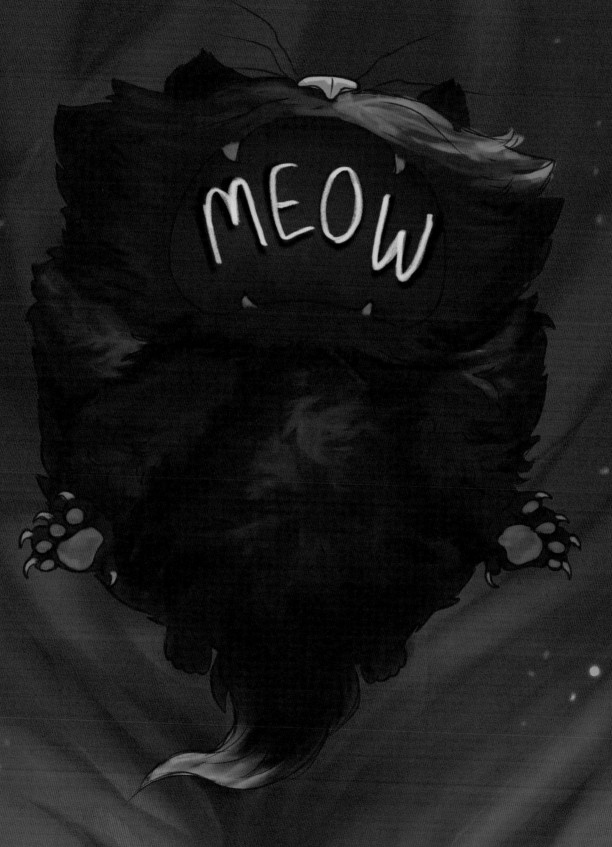

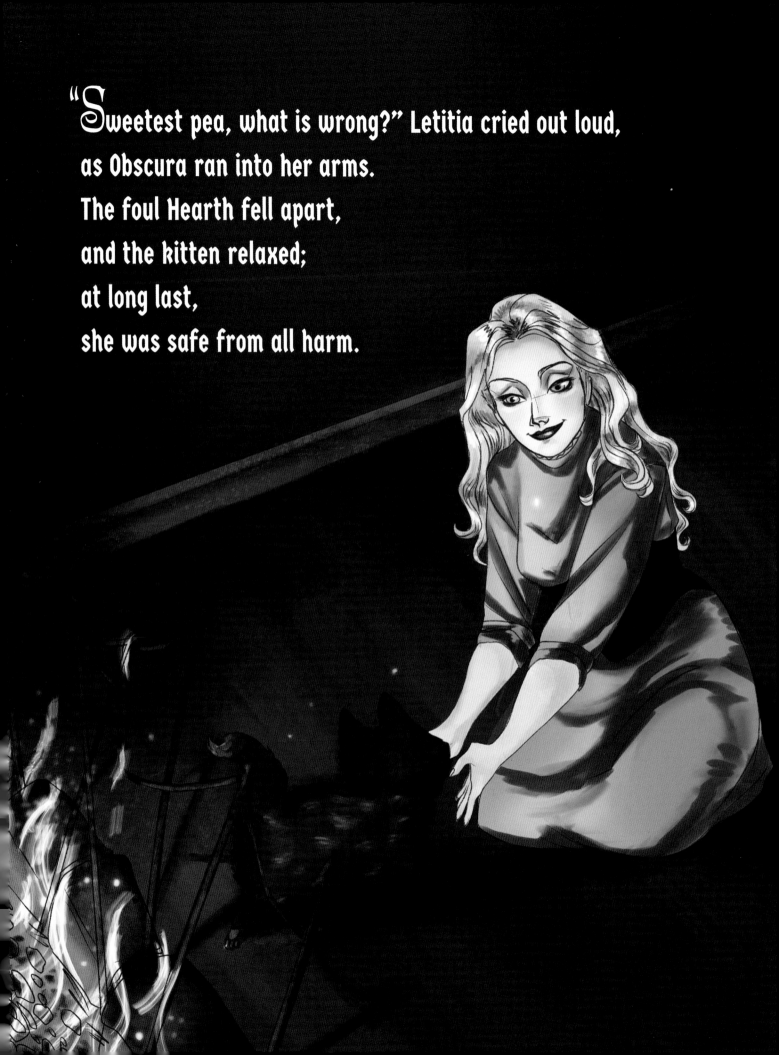

"Sweetest pea, what is wrong?" Letitia cried out loud,
as Obscura ran into her arms.
The foul Hearth fell apart,
and the kitten relaxed;
at long last,
she was safe from all harm.

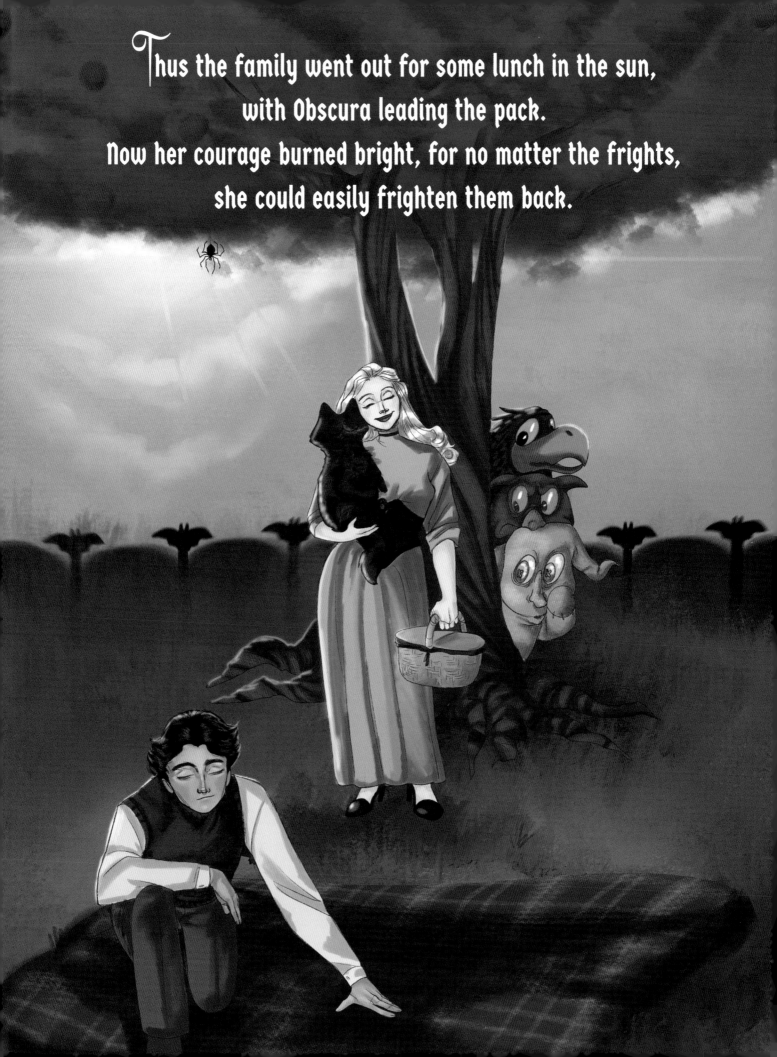

Thus the family went out for some lunch in the sun,
with Obscura leading the pack.
Now her courage burned bright, for no matter the frights,
she could easily frighten them back.

About the Author

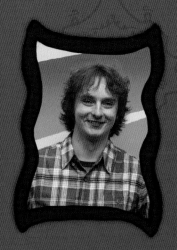

Ben Franchi is a writer based out of Boston, Massachusetts. With an enthusiasm for literature, starting from high school and continuing through his time at Emerson College, Ben has always enjoyed observing the creative possibilities that are hidden throughout everyday life.

Born in Winchester, MA, Ben was an aficionado for the strange and fantastic at a young age, a passion he has taken care to harbor throughout the years. An avid reader from a young age, Ben is constantly on the lookout for the next good book and is a fan of pretty much anything and everything put to print. When he's not traveling the backroads of Concord or taking photographs of the sunset, he enjoys reading about folk history, abstract art, and creative applications of architecture.

About the Illustrator

Cheyenne Bigham always had a passion for art, from childhood all the way to college where she majored in art at the University of North Georgia. Her interests lie in visual storytelling with graphic novels, animation, stop motion animation, sculpting, puppetry, and illustration. Cheyenne was heavily influenced by the films and TV she grew up with and creators like Jim Henson and Guillermo del Toro. Deciding to pursue her interest outside of education, she started with commission work and slowly built a portfolio of personal and commissioned art. Combining her interest in the unusual, whimsical, and her experiences of living in Georgia and Louisiana, she became more inspired by southern gothic imagery and aesthetics. She used this and her love of the kitschy vintage style in the majority of her art.

portrait hall

drawing room

guest room 1

dining room

hall

First